Y0-DOK-877

Quick Keto Meal Prep Cookbook

A Guidebook to Easy Keto Living by Meal Prepping and Tasty Low Carb Ketogenic Diet Recipes (Weight Loss & Time-saving)

By Travis Zehren

© **Copyright 2018 - Travis Zehren -All rights reserved.**

In no way is it legal to reproduce, duplicate, or transmit any part of this document by either electronic means or in printed format. Recording of this publication is strictly prohibited, and any storage of this material is not allowed unless with written permission from the publisher. All rights reserved.

The information provided herein is stated to be truthful and consistent, in that any liability, regarding inattention or otherwise, by any usage or abuse of any policies, processes, or directions contained within is the solitary and complete responsibility of the recipient reader. Under no circumstances will any legal liability or blame be held against the publisher for any reparation, damages, or monetary loss due to the information herein, either directly or indirectly.

Respective authors own all copyrights not held by the publisher.

Legal Notice:
This book is copyright protected. This is only for personal use. You cannot amend, distribute, sell, use, quote or paraphrase any part or the content within this book without the consent of the author or copyright owner. Legal action will be pursued if this is breached.

Table of Contents

Introduction

A number of years ago, I remember that I began to have some health problems that no doctor could identify. I felt sluggish and without energy, especially after I ate. Even though I was eating three solid meals a day, I always felt hungry and undernourished. This led me to snacking throughout the day, mostly with foods that simply were not healthy.

Like most of my peers, my diet was pretty traditional. I would go to the grocery store every weekend and fill up my cart with whatever was on the shelves. White bread for toast in the morning and a sandwich with processed ham for lunch. Spaghetti, white rice, potatoes, pretty much every type of high carb food that you can imagine was a regular staple of my diet.

After several years of feeling generally unhealthy, a friend of mine told me that I should consider trying out a new diet that he had been on for a couple months. When I asked him what foods I would have to give up, he told me that I could eat all the meat and cheese that I wanted. Needless to say that I was interested from the start. When he told me that I would have to give up my morning toast, and those quick spaghetti dinners, however, I wasn't sure what to make of it.

Fast forward seven years later and I can truly say that making the switch to the Keto Diet was the absolute best choice I have ever made. While I made the transition to a full Keto/Low-Carb diet, when I finally did achieve ketosis (after about two weeks) something clicked in my body. I felt more alive, healthier, and my energy levels went through the roof. At work, even my boss (who I despised) noticed an increase in my work production. My increased energy levels motivated me to start taking night classes, and a couple years later, I was able to get my Master's Degree, leave behind the job (and the boss) that I disliked, and start up my own company.

While some people might laugh at the idea that simply cutting out carbs was the key to this whole life transformation, it is fairly easy for me to pinpoint the moment when my life changed. I have been on the Keto Diet for over seven years now, and I think that it is finally time for me to share some of my insights and ideas to help others make the change in their diet. While there certainly is no magic potion to help you overcome all of the obstacles in your life, increased awareness and energy levels are tools that will help you to find the strength you need to make the needed changes yourself.

I truly believe that a low-carb, Keto diet can help people find the motivation to overcome obstacles in life, whatever they may be. In this guidebook, I want to take on the challenge of explaining the basics of the Ketogenic Diet.

The first section will take an in-depth look at some of the basics ideas and terminology of the Keto Diet. Since not everyone has a lot of time when it comes to preparing meals, chapter two looks at some ideas to stay on the Keto Diet even if you are limited in time. Chapter three is simply a list of some of the foods and beverages that you can and cannot eat on the Keto Diet. The last six chapters offer 55 quick and easy Keto recipes that will help you avoid high carb intake without spending hours in the kitchen.

By the end of this book I truly hope that you will be able to discover the changes that are possible by embracing the Keto Diet. Good luck!

Chapter 1: Ketogenic Diet Essentials You Must Know

WHAT IS KETO EXACTLY?

So what exactly is this Keto Diet? That is the first question on every one´s mind. Unfortunately, there are literally thousands of self-proclaimed health gurus in the world of nutrition today, all offering supposed magical diets that will cure all of your problems. The Keto Diet, unlike several other diets out there, is based completely on scientific research.

A Keto Diet is essentially a low carbohydrate diet. IN today´s world, an average man takes in about 296 grams of carbohydrates each day while the average woman consumes around 225 grams of carbohydrates on a daily basis. A diet that is high in carbohydrates will cause your body to produce glucose (for energy) and insulin (to regulate that glucose).

The Keto Diet on the other hand, aims to radically reduce the amount of carbs in our daily diet. In optimum scenarios, people would limit their carb intake to around 20-40 grams per day. While carbohydrates are often considered the part of food that gives your body energy, after 48-72 hours of strictly limiting your carb intake to around the amount listed above, your body will naturally begin to produce a substance known as ketones in the livers. These ketones are an alternative energy source for your body, and the Keto Diet rests on the assumption that fueling your body with ketones rather than with the glucose that is produced through carbohydrate intake offers numerous health benefits that we will explore below.

Is Keto Diet Right for Me?

Unlike other diets that come with a list of who can and cannot participate, the Keto Diet is a great option for the majority of people who want to lose weight, gain energy, and feel generally better. The Keto Diet is specifically recommended for people who are overweight and obese. While there are other low carb diets for weight loss, the Keto diet is unique in that also encourages you to eat foods that are high in beneficial fats. A diet where you can still enjoy steak and cheese is one that most people will enjoy.

The Keto diet might not be a great fit for certain people with unique health issues, including:

- Intolerance to high fat foods (even though the Keto Diet stresses healthy fats)
- People who have had their gall bladder removed
- A history of gallstones
- Fluctuating issues with diabetes or your blood sugar levels

Macronutrients Targets

A Keto diet essentially aims to change your dietary regime so that it is high in fat, moderate (but adequate) in protein and extremely low in carbohydrates. When you compare this "formula" to the food pyramid that has been published by the USDA for decades, the Keto Diet essentially is turning the pyramid on its head. When I first heard of the Keto diet, I remember a feeling of consternation. After years of having been taught that carbohydrates should be the foundation of all diet and that we had to limit our intake of fats and oils, I finally came across a diet that was telling me the exact opposite.

In general, the macronutrient ratios for a Keto diet go as follows:

- 60-75% of calories from fat (more is also possible)

- 15-30% of calories from protein, and
- 5-10 % of calories from carbs.

For example, for a 175 pounds man in his mid-30´s needing around 2000 calories per day, he would need 171 grams of fat (equivalent to around 1500 calories), 92 grams of protein (equivalent to about 350 calories), and 25 grams of carbs (or about 100 calories).

WHAT ARE THE HEALTHY FATS?

Let´s be clear about one thing: just because you decide to start on the Keto diet doesn't mean that you are going to be able to enjoy deep fried foods and other junk food that is extremely high in bad fats. Rather, the Keto Diet stresses eating high amounts of healthy fats. When I started on the Keto diet, I remember vaguely understanding that there was a difference between eating a salad with olive oil as compared to smothering a salad with the commercial Ranch dressing. My grandparents were from Italy, and I remember that during family vacations almost all foods were smothered in a healthy dose of olive oil. Unlike our traditional American fatty diet, however, I distinctly remember feeling better and healthier during those summer vacations.

Healthy fats are sourced from plant-based foods and oils along with oils from certain types of animals (such as fish oil). Healthy fats are needed by your body and can actually radically reduce the risk of heart disease through lowering. Furthermore, healthy fats also can actually lower your blood cholesterol levels through being high in high-density lipoproteins (HDL cholesterol) which is good for you. Among the healthy fats, omega-3 fatty acids have been scientifically proven to promote heart health, weight loss, and other health benefits.

THE AMAZING BENEFITS OF SATURATED FATS

Despite what you learned in your high school nutrition class, saturated fats can be good for you when you choose carefully the source of those fats. The French fries that are deep fried in corn or soybean oil, for example, are much different from the healthy fats found in olive oil, avocadoes, cheeses, nuts, and other types of foods that are promoted on the Keto Diet.

Some of the proven health benefits of saturated fats include:

- Raising levels of HDL cholesterol (the good cholesterol)
- Lowering risk of heart disease
- Lowering the risk of stroke
- Add nutrition to a diet
- Can promote weight loss.

WATCH OUT FOR THE HIDDEN CARBS

One of the biggest challenges for me when starting the Keto diet was that I didn´t realize that there were carbohydrates hiding in so many different types of foods. One of the reasons that it took me so long to actually achieve ketosis is because I didn´t do enough research into where carbohydrates were hiding. While I knew that I was going to have get rid of my white bread that was a staple of my previous unhealthy diet, I didn´t do enough research to where carbohydrates were lurking in dozens of other different foods.

Believe it or not, but carbohydrates can be found in all sorts of different types of food. For example, the garlic powder that I was using to season my meats actually has 6 grams of carbs while oregano have around 3.3 grams. I also thought that the protein bar that I took with me to my morning workout was safe for a Keto diet when it actually had around 7 grams. Lastly, while I knew that dairy products were generally good for the Keto Diet, the slim milk that I was drinking in the mornings was actually contributing carbs to my diet without my knowledge. In general, the amount of carbs in dairy products increases when the fat content is lowered. When I eventually switched to whole milk, the problem was solved.

While it can be frustrating to discover a meal routine that avoids all of these hidden sources of carbohydrates, after a couple weeks you learn to decipher what foods are good for the Keto diet and those that are not.

PROBLEMS WITH OVER CONSUMING CARBS

Unfortunately, our industrial food system has completely ruined the carbohydrates that we eat. While our grandparents probably ate whole grains that they grew on their farms, today's food system is filled with empty, processed carbs and foods that are high in sugars. This is a recipe for disaster. The Keto diet has discovered, however, that even diets that are high in unprocessed, supposedly health carbs comes with a consequence.

High carb diets give you a short boost of energy through the quick production of glucose but will often leave you feeling exhausted and fatigued during the long run once your body uses up the glucose. This can also lead to feelings of hunger causing you to eat more often and thus gain weight. Furthermore, excess carbohydrates in your diet can cause your blood sugar levels to skyrocket. Since most of us live sedentary lifestyles, many of the carbs that we eat are simply not converted to energy, and end up as excess glucose in our body. The high incidence of diabetes can be contributed in part to high carb diets and sedentary lifestyles.

Lastly, high carb diets can lead to obesity which increases the risk of several types of cancer.

How to Calculate Your Proper Carbs Intake

When I first started on the Keto diet, I remember reading columns that tried to help me understand how to read the nutrition labels on the foods I purchased. The problem, of course, is that all of those numbers, percents, and recommended daily values can be pretty confusing to a novice. So how exactly do you go about calculating your proper carb intake to make sure that you are only getting between 5 and 10 percent of your calories from carbs?

For me, the easiest way to calculate my carbs was through using a simple online Keto calculator. There are several of these tools online that you can use for free. By inputting my age, weight, and other basic information, these calculators told me an estimated amount of carbs that I needed to be consuming on a daily basis. Once I had that information, all I needed was to take the time to do some basic calculations.

For example, at the beginning of my Keto journey, I was consuming around 30 grams of carbs per day. By reading the nutrition labels of packaged and canned foods, I was able to determine how many carbs were in each serving size. For fresh fruits, vegetables, dairy products, and meats, all that was needed was a simple Google search to determine how many carbs were in each food. While you might be thinking that this is a lot of work, it was actually a fun learning experience and it became a challenge to discover foods that allowed me to stay under the 30 grams of carbohydrates threshold.

What about Protein Consumption?

Protein is often forgotten part of the Keto diet. While people focus on foods that are high in fat and low in carbs, the focus on moderate protein intake is often overlooked. In our bodies, proteins are known as the building blocks as they help us build and repair tissues. We also need protein to make enzymes, hormones, and other body chemicals. Thus, protein is known as the building block of bones, muscles, cartilage, skin, and blood.

In general, a healthy protein consumption in a Keto diet would be at moderate levels. One easy way to measure this is through aiming to stay or below one gram of protein per day per kilogram of body weight. For example, I weigh about 75 kg, so 75 grams of protein per day is more than enough for me.

MOST USEFUL TIPS FOR THE KETO JOURNEY

One of the things that I wished I'd read when starting on my own Keto journey was a list of some of the top tips. While there is a wealth of information on macronutrient targets, how to achieve Ketosis, etc., sometimes, some simple tips are also needed. Thus, here are five tips from my own Keto Journey:

1. Don't try to achieve ketosis on the first week. Lowering your carb intake gradually is perfectly fine.
2. The Keto diet is more of a lifestyle change rather than a quick fix. Again, make the changes slowly and don't focus on short term goals.
3. During the first months, make it a priority to research the foods you prepare. While this might seem tedious at first, in the long run it will get easier and the more information you have, the easier it will be.
4. Develop a meal plan that you like. Fortunately, with the Keto diet this isn't hard to do as you can eat all the meat and cheese you want.
5. Lastly, use the online tools to help you calculate what you are eating. These tools are free and certainly helpful.

THE UNWANTED SYMPTOMS DURING KETO DIET

After two weeks of having started on the Keto Diet, I remember feeling completely down, as if I had the flu. As with any major dietary change, switching to the Keto diet can lead to a condition known as the Keto flu. This is essentially a collection of symptoms that happen as your body adapts to a low carb diet. Some of the most common symptoms include nausea, constipation, headaches, fatigue and sugar cravings. Not everyone will develop these symptoms, however, and they can be simply avoided through transitioning slowly into the Keto diet. For example, instead of lowering your carb intake from 1,500 grams per day to 20 grams, consider lowering in increments over the period of a month or two so that your body can gradually adapt.

THE BENEFITS OF BEING KETO-ADAPTED

Being Keto-adapted simply means transitioning from relying on glucose (from carbs) for energy to using ketones (from fats) for energy. Our bodies are naturally adapted to produce ketones for reserve energy. Some historians believe that this is a survival instinct that our ancestors developed to help cope during times of famine. However, once your body is regularly producing ketones to deliver the energy you need, there are several benefits.

There are dozens of benefits of becoming Keto adapted. A few of the most important benefits include:

- Increased brain function, memory, and cognitive ability
- Weight loss
- Lower blood sugar
- Increased mitochondrial (cellular) function in the body
- More energy

- More endurance for athletes

HOW TO KEEP KETOSIS IN OPTIMUM LEVEL

Experts recommend ketosis levels that range between 1.5 to 3.0 mmol/l, or milimoles per liter. Lightly nutritional ketosis is defined as anywhere between 0.5 and 1.5 mmol/l. Unless you are a doctor or are regularly doing blood work, these numbers probably don´t mean anything to you. The best way to achieve these specific targets to enjoy the maximum benefits of ketosis, is to stay within your macronutrient levels outlined above. On an anecdotal level, I can tell you from personal experience that after several months of being on the Keto diet, you will simply be able to "feel" when you´re at an optimum Ketosis.

I remember during one business trip, I didn´t plan ahead to bring my own food, and my carbohydrate intake spiked do to a lack of food options. Immediately, I began to feel different as my body switched to using glucose for energy. Even though I didn´t have a way to measure the exact ketone levels in my blood, I am sure that I was not in optimum levels during that trip.

COMMON MISTAKES TO BE AVOIDED

Here is a short list of some of the most common mistakes that I made during the first weeks of being on the Keto diet.

- I didn't pay enough attention to my macronutrient levels. In my case, this led to a reduced amount of protein that was bordering on unhealthy.
- At first, I loved having access to all the meat. However, I probably didn't eat enough of the vegetables recommended on the Keto diet, especially the leafy greens that are important sources of fiber and needed vitamins.

- Obsessing over ketone levels. When you first start on the Keto diet, achieving ketosis is kind of like achieving nirvana. It´s a goal that you absolutely want to achieve. However, obsessing over anything is rarely helpful, and in my case it lead to too much stress.
- Avoid low-fat dairy. If you are going to enjoy dairy, make sure that it is the whole type. As we mentioned above, the lower the fat content in dairy products, the more carbs that are most likely present.

FORMULATING A KETO DIET FOR WEIGHT LOSS

For thousands of people, the main attraction of the Keto diet is that it allows you to meet and sustain weight loss goals. One of the problems of other diets is that quick weight loss is often re-gained in the short term. The Keto diet, on the other hand, allows you to meet your weight loss goals and sustain them in the long run. Furthermore, instead of limiting fat intake and prohibiting you from eating some of your favorite foods, the Keto diet actually encourages more fat intake meaning that you can be on a "diet" and still enjoy chocolate and steak.

By staying within the recommended macronutrient levels, you can also reduce cravings which are a major challenge for people seeking to lose weight.

Lastly, almost all diets also recommend regular exercise to meet and sustain weight loss goals. On the Keto diet, prioritizing low-intensity aerobic exercises will make sure that your body uses fats as the primary energy source.

USING EXERCISE EFFECTIVELY IN A KETO LIFE

One common myth is that you cannot build muscle without excess carbs in your diet. For bodybuilders and others who enjoy time in the gym, you can continue to meet your goals while being on the Keto diet. While I'm not big into hitting the weights, I do jog regularly and I can honestly say that being on the Keto diet hasn't affected my exercise routine. A friend of mine on the Keto diet who is also into bodybuilding, however, tells me that he is able to build muscle mass through moderately increasing his protein intake. Furthermore, his training routine focuses specifically on promoting hypertrophy in his muscles.

A limited carb intake will most likely affect exercise performance if you need high intensity energy levels for specific sports. For example, if you play soccer or other sports without regular stoppages, your performance levels might dip. Furthermore, if you are trying to "max out" in the gym, a lack of carbs might affect your performance. One way to get around this issue you might consider eating a high amount of carbs shortly before the high intensity exercise.

For example, I used to play in a recreational soccer league. To make up for the lack of glucose energy in my body, I would eat a few granola bars (equivalent to about 30 grams of carbs) immediately before playing. This would give me an extra boost of quick energy and actually wouldn't affect my ketosis as I essentially burned off all the excess glucose during the 90 minute soccer game.

SOME FREQUENTLY ASKED QUESTIONS

This first chapter has attempted to answer some of the most common questions that might come up. Because the Keto diet so radically diverges from traditional nutritional suggestions, it can be surprising to read of a diet that recommends high fat intake and strictly limiting carb intake. Below, we offer a quick rundown on some of the most important frequently asked questions.

What does the Keto Diet do?

The Keto diet is designed to help the body achieve a state of nutritional ketosis essentially meaning that your body will burn its fat stores instead of sugars. Once in ketosis, your body does not depend on insulin or glucose to regulate energy levels.

What Can I Eat On The Keto Diet?

While the shopping list for everyone on the Keto diet will be slightly different, it most likely you're your diet will shift to include large doses of meat, fish, eggs, oils, nuts, non-starchy vegetables, leafy greens, and the occasional low-carb fruit. Dairy products and certain types of seeds are also recommended.

What Are The Health Benefits Of The Keto diet?

You can reduce sugar cravings, lose weight, stabilize blood sugar levels, lower blood pressure, reduce inflammation in the body, decrease risk for autoimmune diseases, and increase your energy levels of mental clarity, among many other expected benefits.

Is it Expensive to Eat on the Keto Diet?

While you might spend a bit more during your weekly trip to the grocery store, most people also radically reduce their overall food budget through cutting back on snack foods. Because a high carb diet delivers quick bouts of energy to the body, many people are often left feeling hungry during the day and thus spend money on snacks that are expensive and nutritionally empty.

What Should I Avoid When On The Keto Diet?

While the list is long, here are a few things that should absolutely be avoided:

- Processed grains like white bread and white rice
- Sugars and artificial sweeteners
- Starchy vegetables like potatoes

- Products made from flour
- Certain types of fruit (though berries in moderation are encouraged)

What Medical Conditions Can This Diet Help With?

The Keto diet is a great option for all different types of people. However, if you have diabetes, a doctor might specifically recommend this diet to you. Furthermore, the Keto diet was originally developed for people suffering from seizures as ketosis can naturally help. Lastly, the anti-inflammatory properties of the Keto diet make it a great option for people suffering from joint problems such as arthritis.

Will I feel a lack of energy without carbs in my diet?

While it is true that carbohydrates give your body energy, your body also have the ability to burn fat to give you energy. Studies have shown that our bodies actually run better when they are burning fat rather than sugar. Many people (myself included) claim that the Keto diet actually increases your energy levels.

I thought it was bad to eat lots of fat?

The Keto diet focuses on the "good" types of fat. Good fats will lower your HDL levels (the bad cholesterol and can actually lower the risk of heart disease.

Chapter 2: Quick Keto Meal Prep Ideas

One of the biggest complaints of people new to the Keto diet is that they fear having to spend large amounts of time learning new tricks in the kitchen. While it is true that the Keto diet will substantially change your diet, after a few weeks you should have a pretty good idea of what can and cannot be eaten. Once you have come up with a list of foods (chapter three offers a complete list of foods and beverages), it is completely possible to develop a fast Keto approach that will allow you to enjoy the benefits of ketosis without spending long hours of your day in the kitchen. This chapter offers eleven useful tips on how to develop a fast Keto approach.

PREPARE YOUR KETO STAPLES IN ADVANCE

With a bit of preparation, you can easily prepare freezer meals for a Keto Diet. After about a year of being on the Keto diet, I left my job to begin the life of an entrepreneur. Needless to say, this obviously cut into the amount of free time I had. To maintain my Keto diet routine, I would spend roughly 3-4 hours each Sunday evening in the kitchen preparing my lunches and dinners ahead of time. I would then put those Keto meals into glass Tupperware and put them in the freezer. Almost all Keto meals can easily be frozen for weeks or months. This means that you simply have to take them out of the freezer, but in the defroster for a few minutes, and then microwave them or heat them up over the stove.

If you don't have room in your freezer, you can also prepare Keto-friendly foods in advance and store them in the refrigerator. For example, you can easily bake or sauté all of your meat products in advance, and leave them covered in the refrigerator to simply heat up in a bit of olive oil or ghee butter.

CHOP AND REFRIGERATE VEGETABLES

Chopping up all of those leafy greens for salads or other meals takes a lot of time. Fortunately, leafy greens can last a long time in the refrigerator. Chopping up all those vegetables and placing them in hermetic Tupperware in the fridge is a great way to reduce the amount of time spent preparing your meals. Lemon or lime juice is Keto-friendly, makes for a great salad dressing, and will also help to keep your leafy greens fresh while in the fridge during the week.

PARBOIL AND FREEZE VEGETABLES

While you could simply purchase frozen and bagged vegetables at the supermarket, fresh vegetables will always have more needed vitamins and minerals. However, cooking fresh vegetables also takes a lot of time. Once you have pre-cut those veggies, consider parboiling them and freezing them. This works especially well for asparagus, radishes, green beans, and other low carb vegetables that aren't very appetizing when eaten raw. The good news is that since potatoes and other root vegetables are not generally consumed in the Keto diet, you will save a lot of time since these vegetables take a notoriously long time to cook.

FREEZE BERRIES AND HERBS

Berries go great with a quick Keto breakfast (see our recipes below), and one way to keep berries preserved is through freezing them. When I went to visit my family in Michigan one year, I picked about a bushel of wild blueberries and strawberries from a local farm and froze them for several months of quick breakfast nutrition. Herbs that you grow in your garden can either be dried out or frozen as well.

MEASURE DRY INGREDIENTS AHEAD OF TIME

I always find it amazing when people can cook without following a recipe. I, on the other hand, need a pretty strict recipe to avoid completely ruining a meal. Instead of bringing out the measuring cup and mini kitchen scale every time I cook, I also spend time on the weekends measuring out dry ingredients into pounds, ounces, and/or cups and tablespoons depending on the new Keto recipes I want to try out that week.

MARINATE FISH AND MEAT OVERNIGHT

Unlike other diets, a Keto diet certainly does not lack in flavor. There are several oils, herbs, and seasonings that are all extremely low in carbs. And since meat, poultry, and seafood are all thumbs up in the Keto diet, I usually experiment with different types of marinades. One way to speed up meal preparation is to marinate your meat, poultry, and seafood meals the night before, or even several days before. In some cases, I even prepare meat dishes several days ahead of time and leave them soaking up the flavor.

MAKE CONDIMENTS FOR YOURSELF

Condiments and dressing that you purchase at the grocery store most likely have added sugars, sweeteners, and other ingredients that will load you up on the carbs. When I started on the Keto diet, I found myself experimenting with my own condiments. A simple combination of vinegar, olive oil, and lemon juice (all Keto-friendly) makes for an excellent salad dressing. Adding any odd combination of herbs is also a great way to add flavor. By pre-preparing the condiments for your meals, you will eventually end up with several glass bottles of delicious flavorings at your fingertips for preparing your Keto meals.

USING PRESSURE COOKER

Pressure cookers or instant pots are also a great tool to have in your Keto-inspired kitchen. These essential tools will allow you to throw some ingredients together and leave them cooking while you focus on other activities during the day. One of my favorite pressure cooker/instant pot recipes is No-noodle lasagna (see recipe below). This delicious low carb meal is made from beef, cheese, and eggs, and tastes just like the real thing without the carbs. What's best is that it can be prepared in just minutes while the Instant Pot does its job.

MAKE BONE BROTH, CHICKEN STOCK OR VEGETABLE STOCK

Broth or stock is one of the liquids/beverages approved by the Keto diet because it is essentially free of carbs. While drinking a glass of cold chicken stock might not sound appetizing, make sure to store your bone broth, chicken stock, or vegetable stock for later use. Since you will most likely be preparing lots of meat on your Keto diet journey, storing the broth and stock for later use means that you can whip up a soup quickly when you're in a hurry.

PURPOSING LEFTOVERS

Lastly, you should always make sure to use the leftovers that are inevitable part of the any food prep. While prepping your food in advance will certainly cut back on food waste, you will most likely always have a good amount of leftovers. Leftover meats can be marinated and make into sandwiches with Keto-bread substitutes to take to work the next day, to name just one example.

With these simple tips, preparing nourishing and healthy Keto recipes can be achieved without spending laborious hours over the stove on a daily basis.

Chapter 3: Quick Keto Food List

Many of the most popular diets out there have long lists of foods that you need to avoid. Fortunately, the Keto diet is more about letting you enjoy some of your favorite foods, rather than focusing on prohibitions. While switching to a low carb diet will certainly force you to get of some of the foods that used to be a common feature in your kitchen, this diet still allows you to choose from a wide variety of foods for a rich and varied diet.

It can certainly be helpful to have a complete list of foods that are both approved and prohibited on the Keto diet. The lists below, then, will function as a quick checklist for people who are new to the Keto diet. We have divided the "what to eat" and "what to avoid" sections into food categories for fast reference.

WHAT TO EAT
Fats & Oils

- Fatty Fish
- Non-hydrogenated animal fats
- Lard
- Tallow
- Avocados
- Egg Yolks
- Macadamia/Brazil Nuts
- Butter/Ghee
- Mayonnaise
- Coconut Butter
- Cocoa Butter
- Olive Oil

- Coconut Oil
- Avocado Oil
- Macadamia Oil
- MCT Oil

Protein

- Fish and shellfish
- Whole eggs
- Beef (grass fed is best)
- Free range poultry
- Pork
- Offal/organs: great source of vitamins and minerals
- Fatty cuts of veal, lamb, venison, etc.
- Nut butters like almond butter

Vegetables

- Leafy greens like spinach and kale
- Cabbage
- Green beans
- Baby Bella Mushrooms
- Bok Choy
- Celery
- Asparagus
- Arugula
- Swiss Chard
- Avocado
- Daikon Radish

Fruits

- Berries are best
- Strawberries
- Raspberries
- Blueberries

- Avocado (actually a fruit)
- Green olives
- Coconut
- Rhubarb
- Carambola (Star fruit)
- Blackberries
- Lemon juice

Dairy

- Almost all dairy products are fine on a Keto diet as long as you opt for whole dairy products, including,
- Yogurt, especially Greek Yogurt that is not artificially sweetened.
- Heavy whipping cream
- Cottage cheese
- Cream cheese
- Sour Cream
- Soft cheese varieties like mozzarella, brie, blue, Colby, Monterey jack, and others
- Hard cheese varieties such as aged cheddar, parmesan, feta, Swiss, and others
- Whole milk

Nuts and Seeds

- Fattier nuts are best like macadamias and almonds
- Brazil nuts
- Pecans
- Hazelnuts and walnuts in moderation

Pseudo-grains and Alternative Flours

- Quinoa and amaranth in moderation
- Flaxseed meal
- Almond Flour
- Coconut Flour

- Chia seed meal

WHAT TO AVOID
Foods high in carbohydrates

- Refined sugars
- Refined wheat products like white bread
- Pastas
- Potatoes and other root vegetables
- Rice in high quantity
- Fish and shellfish

Vegetables

- Potatoes and sweet potatoes
- Corn
- Beets
- Squash and pumpkin
- Carrots
- Onions
- Parsnips
- Leeks
- Green peas

Fruits

- Apples
- Starchy fruits like bananas and plantains
- Most other sweet fruits with the exception of berries are usually on the "no-eat" list due to the carbs present in the naturally occurring sugars.

Dairy

- Low Fat milk

- "Light" cheese products
- Super sweet yogurt
- Cream cheese has one of the highest carb ratings among dairy products so should be consumed in moderation

Nuts and Seeds

- Pistachios and cashews are both very high in carbs and should be avoided

Other Foods to Avoid

- Cheap oils made from palm oil or soybean oil
- Processed meats that might contain artificial sweeteners (like bacon and lunch meat)

SOME BEVERAGE IDEAS

- Water is always okay
- Naturally flavored water, such as with lemon juice
- Tea
- Coffee
- Almond milk
- Coconut milk
- Soup Broth
- Club soda
- Hemp milk

Chapter 4: Top 20 Keto Breakfast and Lunches

EGG CUPS

Serves: 4

Preparation time: 15 minutes

Ingredients:

- 4 eggs
- 1 cup onion, diced
- 1 cup bell pepper, diced
- 1 cup mushrooms, diced
- 1 cup tomatoes, diced
- ½ cup cheddar cheese, shredded
- ¼ cup half and half
- Salt and pepper to taste
- 2 tablespoons cilantro, chopped

Preparation:

- Combine all the ingredients in a bowl.
- Divide the mixture into 4 glass jars.
- Put on the lids but do not close tightly.
- Pour 2 cups of water into the Instant Pot.
- Place a steamer rack inside the pot.
- Put the jars on top of the rack.
- Cover the pot.
- Set it to manual.
- Cook at high pressure for 5 minutes.
- Release the pressure quickly.

Serving Suggestion: You can also set aside some cheese and use it for topping.

Tip: Use different colored bell peppers to make the dish colorful.

Nutritional Information per Serving:

- Calories   173
- Total Fat 16g
- Saturated Fat 8.4g
- Cholesterol 184mg
- Sodium 161mg
- Total Carbohydrate 6.5g
- Dietary Fiber 1.8g
- Total Sugars 4.6g
- Protein 11.1g
- Potassium 356mg

Sausage Balls with Cheese

Serves: 2-3

Preparation time: 25 minutes

Ingredients:

- 20 ounces pork sausage for breakfast
- 2 ounces cheddar cheese,
- 20 small cubes of cheddar cheese
- Fat for frying

Preparation: Remove the sausage meat the skins and mix in the grated cheese. Take the individual cubes of cheddar cheese and hand mold the meat mixture around the cubes into small balls. Heat the fat in a skillet and fry the sausage balls until browned on all sides.

Serving Suggestion: This hearty is best served warm.

Nutritional Information per Serving:

- Calories 189
- Fat 16.9g
- Carbohydrate 0.4g
- Dietary Fiber 0g
- Net Carbs 0.4g
- Protein 8.9g

HEARTY EGGS AND BEEF BREAKFAST

Serves: 3-4

Preparation time: 20 minutes

Ingredients:

- 1 pound minced beef (not too lean)
- 6 large eggs
- 10 medium cloves of garlic
- Paprika powder

Preparation: Hard boil the eggs. Crush or very finely chop the garlic and mix with the minced beef. Divide into 6 portions. Make a patty and mold the meat and garlic mixture around each egg. Grill or bake these eggs until cooked.

Serving Suggestion: Once cooked, cut these in half and serve sprinkled with the paprika.

Nutritional Information per Serving:

- Calories 319
- Fat 13.3g
- Carbohydrate 0.7g
- Dietary Fiber 0g
- Net Carbs 0.7g
- Protein 46.5g

CHICKEN AND BACON WRAPS

Serves: 3-4

Preparation time: 35 minutes

Ingredients:

- 1.5 pounds of chicken fillets
- 12 bacon strips

Preparation: Pre-heat the oven to 375°F and cover a baking tray with aluminum foil. Cut the fillets and bacon strips into 25 pieces. Wrap a piece of bacon around each piece of chicken and then on the foil lined tray with the bacon facing downwards. Bake for about 25minutes until brown and the bacon is crisp. Drain the excess fat away on a paper towel before serving.

Serving Suggestion: Place a cocktail stick in chicken wrap and serve with a simple tomato sauce for dipping.

Nutritional Information per Serving:

- Calories 59
- Fat 2.8g
- Carbohydrate 0g
- Dietary Fiber 0g
- Net Carbs 0g
- Protein 8.1g

PEPPERONI PIZZA ON A CHEESE BASE/CRUST

Serves: 3-4

Preparation time: 40 minutes

Ingredients:

- 8 ounces mozzarella cheese, shredded
- Garlic seasoning
- Italian herb seasoning or herbs of your choice
- 2 ounces pepperoni, chopped

Preparation: Heat a large skillet over a medium heat and then sprinkle in the cheese to completely cover the base. Add garlic, pepperoni, and herb seasoning when the cheese starts to bubble. When the edges of the pizza begin to brown and it begins to loosen from the bottom of the skillet, slide the pizza out onto a serving plate.

Serving Suggestion: This pizza doesn't have the traditional cheese sauce, but you could serve as pizza sauce infused with rosemary, oregano, and basil for the slices to be dipped into while eating.

Nutritional Information per Serving:

- Calories 241
- Fat 17.6g
- Carbohydrate 2.2g
- Dietary Fiber 0g
- Net Carbs 2.2g
- Protein 17.9g

EGG AND SAUSAGE BURGER

Serves: 4

Preparation time: 25 minutes

Ingredients:

- 1 pound pork breakfast sausage meat
- 4 large fresh farm eggs
- 2 tbsp. olive oil
- 2 tsp. fresh herbs of your choice
- Salt and Pepper
- Hot chili sauce (optional)

Preparation: In a small bowl mix the sausage meat with the herbs and season to taste. Divide the sausage into 8 portions and flatten into a patty. Heat olive oil and fry the patty on both sides until evenly cooked. Remove and drain excess grease. Fry the eggs either sunny side up or scrambled and serve between the sausage patties which serve as the bun.

Serving Suggestion: If you want a breakfast with a kick, top the burger with a bit of the optional chili sauce.

Nutritional Information per Serving:

- Calories 419
- Fat 35.2g
- Carbohydrate 3.0g
- Dietary Fiber 1.0 g
- Net Carbs 2.0g
- Protein 24.7g

A Light Salmon Lunch

Serves: 3-4

Preparation time: 25 minutes

Ingredients:

- 2 pounds fresh salmon
- 8 ounces smoked salmon
- 2 fresh eggs
- ½ cup almond flour
- 2 tsp. soy sauce
- 1 tbsp. chopped green onions
- 2 cloves garlic
- Salt and pepper to taste
- Oil for frying

Preparation: Skin and bone the fresh salmon and cut finely. Break the smoked salmon into pieces. In a separate bowl, mix the fish, eggs, almond flour, soy sauce and the rest of the ingredients. Form into 30 evenly sized balls. Fry until brown with a minimal amount of oil. Garnish with parsley and serve with lemon wedges.

Serving Suggestion: Make sure that the smoked salmon you purchase is NOT sugar smoked to avoid adding extra carbs to this meal.

Nutritional Information per Serving:

- Calories 60
- Fat 3.4g
- Carbohydrate 0.2g
- Dietary Fiber 0g
- Net Carbs 0.2g
- Protein 7.3g

CHEDDAR PANCAKES: A BREAKFAST DELIGHT

Serves: 4

Preparation time: 30 minutes

Ingredients:

- 4 large egg whites
- 2 cups almond meal
- 4 ounces cheddar cheese,
- 2 tbsp. green onion, finely chopped
- 2 cloves garlic, finely chopped
- 1 tsp. baking powder
- 4 tbsp. olive oil
- ½ cup water
- Oil to grease a skillet

Preparation: Mix all of the ingredients in a bowl. Use just a bit of oil on the skillet or non-stick frying pan. Pour a bit of the pancake batter and cook until bubbles rise to the surface. Turn with a spatula and cook for about one more minute.

Serving Suggestion: While these aren't necessarily a sweet pancake, a simple fruit jam made from berries and sweetened with stevia extract offers an interesting blend of flavors.

Nutritional Information per Serving:

- Calories 210
- Fat 19.5g
- Carbohydrate2.5g
- Dietary Fiber 0.8g
- Net Carbs 1.7g
- Protein 8.2g

Smoked Salmon with an Oriental Twist

Serves: 3-4

Preparation time: 45 minutes

Ingredients:

- 12 ounces smoked salmon (without sugar)
- 2 cucumbers
- 1 avocado
- 7 ounces cream cheese
- Wasabi to taste
- ¼ cup sesame seeds
- ½ cup soy sauce for dip

Preparation: Beat the cream cheese with a little wasabi paste until smooth. Lay out the smoked salmon on waxed paper and spread with cream cheese. Cut the avocado and cucumber and lay next to the salmon. With the waxed paper roll up the salmon from vegetable end. Add sesame seeds and cut each roll into one inch portions. Serve with soy sauce and ginger.

Serving Suggestion: These little bites gather flavor the longer you leave them in the refrigerator so consider preparing ahead of time and letting sit overnight.

Nutritional Information per Serving:

- Calories 156
- Fat 11.8g
- Carbohydrate 5.4g
- Dietary Fiber 1.9g
- Net Carbs 4.1g
- Protein 8.2g

TUNA AND SEAWEED ROLLS

Serves: 3

Preparation time: 30 minutes

Ingredients:

- 2 sheets of dried seaweed
- 2 cans tuna fish
- 4 tbsp. mayonnaise
- 4 tbsp. parsley, finely chopped
- 1 medium ripe avocado cut into slices
- ¼ red sweet bell pepper, finely sliced
- Chili sauce

Preparation: Mix the tuna, mayonnaise and parsley. Lay out the dried seaweed (a sushi mat helps a lot if you have one). Spread the tuna mixture over the dried seaweed and add the pepper and avocado slices. Roll up and press firmly so that the dried seaweed sticks together. Cut into pieces and serve with chili on top.

Serving Suggestion: Nori seaweed rolls are the best for this recipe, though you can use other types.

Nutritional Information per Roll:

- Calories 118
- Fat 7.6g
- Carbohydrate 2.8g
- Dietary Fiber 1.4g
- Net Carbs 1.4g
- Protein 9.4g

NUTTY MUSHROOMS

Serves: 3

Preparation time: 40 minutes

Ingredients:

- 12 mushroom caps
- ¾ cup walnut or macadamia pieces
- 1 cup chopped parsley
- 3 cloves garlic, finely chopped
- ¼ cup grated parmesan cheese
- ¼ cup olive oil
- 12 slices mozzarella cheese
- Salt and pepper to taste

Preparation: Place the mushrooms on a broiler pan with the top side down. Mix in a food processor and then add the olive oil until a paste is formed. Place this paste inside the mushroom caps and top with a slice of mozzarella cheese. Place under the broiler for 7 minutes or until the cheese is bubbling.

Serving Suggestion: This makes a great and filling lunch alongside a simple salad.

Nutritional Information per Serving:

- Calories 160
- Fat 14.1g
- Carbohydrate2.2g
- Dietary Fiber 1.0g
- Net Carbs 1.2g
- Protein 8.2g

Zucchini Breakfast Hash

Serves: 2

Preparation time: 35 minutes

Ingredients:

- 1 medium zucchini
- 2 slices bacon
- ½ small white onion or 1 clove garlic
- 1 tbsp. ghee or coconut oil
- 1 tbsp. freshly chopped parsley or chives
- ¼ tsp. salt
- 1 large egg on top or ½ medium avocado

Preparation: Peel and chop the onion (or garlic) and slice the bacon. Cook the onion over a medium heat and add the bacon. Cut the zucchini into medium pieces and add the zucchini to the pan and cook for 10-15 minutes. When done, remove from the heat and add chopped parsley. Top with a fried egg or avocado.

Serving Suggestion: This wholesome breakfast is complete and you can add both the egg and the avocado if you'd like.

Nutritional Information per Serving:

- Total carbs: 9.1g
- Fiber 2.5g
- Net carbs 6.6g
- Protein 17.4 g
- Fat 35.5 g
- Calories 422 kcal
- Magnesium 53 mg
- Potassium 775 mg

All Day Breakfast

Serves: 1

Preparation time: 15 minutes

Ingredients:

- 1 large egg
- 5 bacon slices
- 2 large Portobello mushrooms
- ½ average avocado
- 1 tbsp. ghee
- pinch freshly ground black pepper
- salt to taste
- fresh herbs for garnish

Preparation: Heat the ghee on a nonstick pan over medium-low heat. Add the mushrooms with salt and pepper and cook for about 7 minutes until tender. Drain the excess water and fry the egg with the bacon.

Serving Suggestion: If you don't like mushrooms, substitute one cup of spinach cooked in olive oil or butter.

Nutritional Information per Serving:

- Total carbs 15.5g
- Fiber 8.9 g
- Net Carbs 6.6g
- Protein 19.5 g
- Fat 41.3 g
- Calories 489 kcal

HERBS AND MUSHROOMS LUNCH

Serves: 3

Preparation time: 25 minutes

Ingredients:

- 10 ounces sautéed mushrooms
- 1 small onion, finely chopped
- 5 ounces cheddar cheese, grated
- 3 large fresh eggs, separated
- ¼ cup chopped dill
- ¼ cup chopped parsley
- 1 tbsp. chopped thyme
- 2 tbsp. olive oil
- Salt and pepper to taste

Preparation: Preheat the oven to 400°F. Fry onions in olive oil and then add mushrooms and herbs. Stir in egg yolks and cheese and season to taste. In separate bowl, beat the egg whites until soft peaks forms and fold them into the mushroom mix. Spoon the mix into a baking tin and cook for 25 minutes. Once cooled cut into slices and serve warm or chilled.

Serving Suggestion: This simple lunch can be prepared ahead of time and kept in the refrigerator for an easy "take-with-you" lunch for folks who have short lunch hours while at work.

Nutritional Information per Serving:

- Calories 144
- Fat 11.8g
- Carbohydrate 3.7g
- Dietary Fiber 1.1g
- Net Carbs 2.6g
- Protein 6.7g.

SMOKED TROUT LUNCH

Serves: 3-4

Preparation time: 45 minutes

Ingredients:

- 4 ounces smoked trout
- 4 ounces cream cheese
- 2 tbsp. onion, grated
- 2 tbsp. lemon juice
- ½ tsp. Worcestershire sauce
- ½ tsp. freshly ground black pepper
- Tabasco to taste
- Chopped chives to garnish
- 1 small cucumber

Preparation: Mix all of the ingredients into a processor or blender and blend until smooth. If it is too thick add more lemon juice. Place spoonfulls onto the cucumber slices and sprinkle with chives for a delightful light lunch.

Serving Suggestion: Consider changing Keto cracker substitutes for the cucumbers for a more filling alternative.

Nutritional Information per Serving:

- Calories 29
- Fat 2.0g
- Carbohydrate 0.8g
- Dietary Fiber 0g
- Net Carbs 0.8g
- Protein 2.0g

SCRAMBLED EGGS WITH PESTO

Serves: 2

Preparation time: 15 minutes

Ingredients:

- 3 large eggs
- 1 tbsp. butter or ghee
- 1 tbsp. pesto
- 2 tbsp. crème fraiche or sour cream or creamed coconut milk
- salt to taste
- freshly ground black pepper to taste

Preparation:

Crack the eggs into a mixing bowl with a pinch of salt and pepper and beat them well with a whisk or fork. Pour the eggs into a pan, add butter or ghee and turn the heat on. Keep on low heat while stirring constantly. Do not stop stirring as the eggs may get dry and lose the creamy texture. Add the pesto and mix in well. Once off the heat, add the crème fraiche in and mix well with the eggs.

Serving Suggestion: Serve with sliced avocado on top.

Nutritional Information per Serving:

- Total Carbs: 3.3g
- Fiber 0.7 g
- Net carbs 2.6 g
- Protein 20.4 g
- Fat 41.5 g
- Calories 467 kcal

CHOCOLATE CHIA PUDDING FOR BREAKFAST!

Serves: 1-2

Preparation time: 15 minutes

Ingredients:

- ¼ cup chia seeds
- ¼ cup coconut milk or heavy whipping cream
- ¼ cup water or almond milk
- ¼ cup pumpkin purée, unsweetened
- 5-10 drops Stevia extract
- ½ tsp. pumpkin pie spice mix

Preparation: Combine the chia seeds, coconut milk, water, pumpkin puree, pumpkin pie spice mix, and the stevia. If you prefer a smoother texture, use ground chia seeds.

Serving Suggestion: You can make a large batch of this early in the week and have a great breakfast smoothie to take with you on your commute to work.

Nutritional Information per Serving:

- Total Carbs: 20.8g
- Fiber 14.2 g
- Net carbs 7.2 g
- Protein 6.6 g
- Fat 8.1 g
- Calories 295 kcal

BERRY AND CHIA PUDDING

Serves: 1-2

Preparation time: 15 minutes

Ingredients:

- ¼ cup chia seeds
- ¼ cup coconut milk or heavy whipping cream
- ½ cup water or almond milk
- ¼ tsp. cinnamon
- 10 drops Stevia extract
- ¼ cup berries, fresh or frozen

Preparation: Mix the chia seeds, coconut milk, water, cinnamon and stevia. If you prefer a smoother texture, place into a blender and pulse until smooth. Mix in the fresh or frozen berries and enjoy

Serving Suggestion: The almond milk will offer a thicker smoothie texture while the water will make it more like a breakfast drink.

Nutritional Information per Serving:

- Total Carbs: 20.3g
- Fiber 14.5 g
- Net carbs 5.8 g
- Protein 7.9 g
- Fat 22.4 g
- Calories 288 kcal

WAFFLES WITH CHEESE

Serves: 2-3

Preparation time: 25 minutes

Ingredients:

- 2 cups raw cauliflower crumbs
- 2 cups grated mozzarella cheese
- ½ cup grated parmesan
- 4 fresh eggs
- 2 tsp. garlic powder
- 2 tsp. onion powder
- 1 tsp. freshly ground black pepper
- 2 tbsp. chopped chives
- Salt to taste
- Butter for greasing

Preparation: Mix all of the ingredients in a bowl. Add a ½ cup of this batter into your hot waffle maker and cook for 4-5 minutes. Remove and cool. You can also cook on a hot griddle if you don't have a waffle maker.

Serving Suggestion: If you like a sweet and salty combination, a bit of elderberry syrup would go great with this filling breakfast.

Nutritional Information per Serving:

- Calories 112
- Fat 7.3g
- Carbohydrate 2.3g
- Dietary Fiber 0.6g
- Net Carbs 1.7g
- Protein 8.9g.

Sushi Rolls—Bacon Style

Serves: 3-4

Preparation time: 20 minutes

Ingredients:

- 1 pound smoky bacon slices
- 4 ounces mozzarella cheese, shredded
- 1 tsp. hot chili sauce

Preparation: Pre-heat the oven to 400°F. Lay the bacon slices on a baking tray and bake until well browned for about 18 minutes. Place the bacon on a mat with the edges of each slice slightly overlapping. Sprinkle with the cheese and hot sauce and roll up as you would with sushi. Place the tray back into the over for 8 minutes to melt the cheese. Remove, let cool, and slice into 12 rolls.

Serving Suggestion: You will want to serve this hot. Accompany with a breakfast drink.

Nutritional Information per Serving:

- Calories 99
- Fat 7.3g
- Carbohydrate 0.4g
- Dietary Fiber 0g
- Net Carbs 0.4g
- Protein 7.1g.

Chapter 5: Top 10 Keto Dinners

LAMB FILLET WITH ROSEMARY AND SPICES

Serves: 2

Preparation time: 35 minutes

Ingredients:

- 1 tbsp.   ground   cumin
- 1 tbsp.   ground   turmeric
- 3 drops   liquid stevia extract (adjust   to taste)
- 1 tbsp.   hazelnut oil (or other nut oil)
- 2 cloves   garlic, crushed
- 1 tbsp.   fresh cilantro, chopped
- ground Salt and   pepper   to season
- 2 pounds lamb fillet
- 1 small   bunch   fresh mint, chopped
- 4 ounces thick plain yogurt
- Vegetable oil for frying
- 20 rosemary stalks

Preparation: Mix together the first seven ingredients in a large bowl and season   to taste. Next, cut the lamb into strips and put in bowl to allow to marinade overnight. After marinating, mix the mint and yogurt. Thread the lamb onto rosemary skewers and fry on high heat in the vegetable oil until evenly browned. Serve with the yogurt and mint dip for a lovely meal.

Serving Suggestion: Sprinkle the yogurt with whole mint leaves for some extra punch.

Tip: You can easily grow your own rosemary outside your home.

Nutritional Information per Serving:

- Calories 108
- Fat 5.1g,
- Carbohydrate 0.8g
- Dietary   Fiber 0g
- Net Carbs 0.8g
- Protein   13.5g

BEEF BALLS WITH SOY AND GINGER

Serves: 4

Preparation time: 30 minutes

Ingredients:

- 1 pound ground beef (turkey burger makes a great option as well)
- 1 finely chopped small onion
- 1 fresh egg
- ½ tsp. salt
- ½ tsp. black pepper
- 2 cloves garlic, minced

To make the sauce, you will also need the following ingredients:

- ¼ cup soy sauce
- 2 tbsp. rice wine vinegar (or sake, if you can find it)
- 1 tbsp. fresh ginger, grated
- 1 tbsp. green onion or chives, chopped
- 1 clove garlic, minced
- 2 drops liquid stevia extract (adjust to taste)

Preparation: Pre-heat the oven to 425°F. Put all of the ingredients into a bowl and mix together with your hands. Shape the meat into small balls about 1. 5 inches in diameter and bake in the oven for about 12 minutes or until brown but not dried out. Check for thorough and complete cooking. Next, mix all of the sauce ingredients. To serve, put 2-3 balls on a cocktail stick and serve around the dipping sauce.

Serving Suggestion: Serve with a side of rice of quinoa and a kale salad.

Nutritional Information per Serving:

- Calories 34
- Fat 1.1g
- Carbohydrate 0.5g
- Dietary Fiber 0g
- Net Carbs 0.5g
- Protein 4.9g

PARMESAN CHICKEN BALLS

Serves: 4

Preparation time: 30 minutes

Ingredients:

- 1.5 pounds ground white chicken,
- 1 cup almond flour
- ½ cup parmesan cheese
- ½ cup full cream milk
- Salt and black pepper
- ½ tsp. dried oregano
- 1 cup marinara sauce
- 3 ounces fresh mozzarella cheese

Preparation: Pre-heat the oven to 375°F. Grease a glass, ovenproof dish and set aside. In a large bowl mix together half of the almond flour, the parmesan cheese, whole milk, seasonings and herbs, and the chicken and stir. Divide into 24 portions and roll into a ball. Rolle in the rest of the almond flour and place in the dish. Bake for 15-20 minutes and then add a spoonful of marinara sauce and slice of mozzarella cheese. Cook for 10 more minutes. Sprinkle with dried oregano and enjoy.

Serving Suggestion: This is a great dinner to be served with a rice pilaf.

Nutritional Information per Serving:

- Calories 72
- Fat 3.1g
- Carbohydrate 2.2g
- Dietary Fiber 0g
- Net Carbs 2.2g
- Protein 8.6g

SALAMI ROLLUPS

Serves: 3

Preparation time: 15 minutes

Ingredients:

- 8 large slices salami
- 8 ounces cream cheese
- ½ cup plain yogurt
- 3 cloves garlic, finely chopped
- A bit of Worcestershire sauce
- Salt and pepper to taste

Preparation: Mix together everything but the salami and divide into nine even portions. Put one portion along the middle of a slice of salami and roll up from one side. Repeat with the rest of the mixture.

Serving Suggestion: Have a bowl of olive oil infused with rosemary for dipping these slices.

Nutritional Information per Serving:

- Calories 170
- Fat 14.6g
- Carbohydrate 3.1g
- Dietary Fiber 0g
- Net Carbs 3.1g
- Protein 6.7g

Ricotta and Bacon "Muffins"

Serves: 3

Preparation time: 35 minutes

Ingredients:

- 10 ounces baby spinach
- 1.5 pounds ricotta cheese
- 2 ounces toasted pine nuts, chopped
- 1 cup grated parmesan
- ½ cup thick plain yogurt
- 2 large fresh eggs
- 7 ounces bacon
- Salt and pepper to taste¿

Preparation: Pre-heat the oven to 350°F. Grease a muffin pan with whole butter. Steam the spinach for one minute, drain and chop finely along with the bacon. Mix all ingredients in a food processor and then spoon into muffin cups and cook for 35 minutes or until brown.

Serving Suggestion: This simple, but filling dinner can be accompanied by a small plate of quinoa or a small green salad.

Nutritional Information per Muffin:

- Calories 228
- Fat 16.2g
- Carbohydrate 4.8g
- Dietary Fiber 0.7g
- Net Carbs 4.1 g
- Protein 16.4g

ROLLS OF ZUCCHINI AND SALMON

Serves: 2-3

Preparation time: 35 minutes

Ingredients:

- 2 medium zucchini
- A 5 ounce can pink or red salmon
- 1 small avocado
- 2 tbsp. mayonnaise
- 1 small chili pepper
- 3 tsp. lime juice
- Salt and pepper
- Paprika or cayenne pepper to garnish

Preparation: Slice the zucchini thinly lengthways using a potato peeler. Drain the salmon and mix with other ingredients. Place a small spoonful of the fish mixture at one end of each zucchini slice and roll it up using a toothpick to secure it. Garnish with salt and pepper. Use a tooth pick to secure the end if necessary and serve immediately

Serving Suggestion: You can switch the salmon for tuna, crab meat, or any other seafood meat you have on hand.

Nutritional Information per Serving:

- Calories 51
- Fat 3.7g
- Carbohydrate 3.0g
- Dietary Fiber 1.2g
- Net Carbs 1.8g
- Protein 2.3g

CHEESE AND CHICKEN TACOS

Serves: 3

Preparation time: 30 minutes

Ingredients:

2 cups grated mozzarella

2 chicken breasts, cooked and shredded

4 tbsp. sour cream

2 green onions, finely chopped

4 tsp. chili salsa

Salt and pepper

Preparation: Pre-heat the oven to 350°F and line a baking tray with parchment paper. Place ½ cup scoops of the cheese on the baking tray and bake until melted and crunchy. When cooled, roll like a wrap and fill with the cooked chicken, onions, salsa, and sour cream.

Serving Suggestion: You can switch the chicken breasts for pork if you want the authentic Mexican "al pastor" taco flavor.

Nutritional Information per Serving:

- Calories 367
- Fat 20.4g
- Carbohydrate 3.3g
- Dietary Fiber 0g
- Net Carbs 3.3g
- Protein 40.6g

CHEESY CHICKEN FINGERS

Serves: 4

Preparation time: 35 minutes

Ingredients:

- 2 pounds chicken breast meat
- 1 cup grated parmesan cheese
- 2 tbsp. chopped herbs, thyme or parsley
- Salt and pepper to taste
- 1 tsp. powdered chili pepper
- 4 ounces butter
- 4 cloves garlic, finely chopped

Preparation: Pre-heat the oven to 350°F and grease a baking sheet with butter. Brown the chopped garlic with butter. Mix the cheese herbs and chili pepper on a plate. Cut the chicken into 20 or so fingers and dip into the cheese mixture. Place on the baking sheet and cook for 25 minutes or until golden brown. Turn halfway through for even cooking.

Serving Suggestion: This meal can be stored in the fridge if you are prepping meals beforehand and can easily be warmed up by microwave while on a quick lunch break.

Nutritional Information per Serving:

- Calories 121
- Fat 6.6g
- Carbohydrate 0.6g
- Dietary Fiber 0g
- Net Carbs 0.6g
- Protein 14.2g

CHINESE CHICKEN WINGS

Serves: 4

Preparation time: 60 minutes

Ingredients:

- 2 pounds chicken wings
- 1 cup soy sauce
- ½ cup water
- ½ tsp. chili oil
- 1 tbsp. sesame oil
- 2 tbsp. lemon juice
- 3 cloves garlic, finely chopped
- 1 tbsp. fresh minced ginger

Preparation: Mix together all of the ingredients and then place the wings in the marinade and let sit overnight. Pre-heat the oven to 375°F. Oil a roasting tin and place the drained wings on it. Cook for 55 minutes and serve either warm or cool.

Serving Suggestion: This tasty dinner goes great with a salad and rice pilaf.

Nutritional Information per Chicken Wing:

- Calories 85
- Fat 3.5g
- Carbohydrate 1.2g
- Dietary Fiber 0g
- Net Carbs 1.2g
- Protein 11.7g

CHEESY PEPPERONI MUFFINS

Serves: 4

Preparation time: 40 minutes

Ingredients:

- 3 ounces ground flax seed
- 1½ tsp. baking powder
- 2 tbsp. Italian seasoning
- 8 fresh eggs, lightly beaten
- 8 ounces mozzarella cheese, shredded
- ½ cup grated parmesan cheese
- 7 ounces pepperoni, finely diced
- Salt and pepper to taste

Preparation: Pre-heat the oven to 375°F and grease 12 muffin cups. Mix together the flax seed, baking powder, Italian seasoning and salt and pepper. Add the beaten eggs along with the cheeses and pepperoni. Spoon into the cups and cook for about 20 minutes.

Serving Suggestion: These Italian-flavored dinner is hearty enough to stand on its own. You can however, combine with a simple salad as well.

Nutritional Information per Serving:

- Calories 254
- Fat 19.1g
- Carbohydrate 4.3g
- Dietary Fiber 2.0g
- Net Carbs 2.3g
- Protein 16.8

Chapter 6: Top 10 Keto Snacks

CUCUMBER AND AVOCADO CROUTES

Serves: 3

Preparation time: 15 minutes

Ingredients:

- 1 cucumber, cut into thin slices
- 8 ounces cream cheese
- 1 large avocado
- Fresh lemon juice to taste
- 3 drops of hot sauce (optional)
- Slices of green onion or chives
- 3 ounce can of salmon, flaked

Preparation: Remove the avocado flesh from the skin and mash it with the cream cheese. Beat well until smooth. Add seasonings including lemon juice and the hot sauce. Add this mixture onto the cucumber slice and top with flaked salmon and some onion or chives. Enjoy! Serving Suggestion:

Nutritional Information per Serving

- Calories 72
- Fat 6.3g
- Carbohydrate 2.3g
- Dietary Fiber 1.0g
- Net Carbs 1.3g
- Protein 2.4g

PARMESAN AND WALNUT WAFERS (CRACKER SUBSTITUTE)

Serves: 2

Preparation time: 10 minutes

Ingredients:

- 1 tbsp. of unsalted butter
- 6 ounces parmesan cheese that is grated finely
- 3 tbsp. chopped walnuts
- Fresh thyme and rosemary

Preparation: Pre-heat the oven to 350°F. Line your baking trays with parchment or wax paper. Mix together the butter and cheese and then fold in the walnuts. Drop large spoonfuls of this mixture onto the trays and sprinkle with thyme and rosemary. Let brown in the oven for 8 minutes. Cool on a wire rack before enjoying.

Serving Suggestion: These go great with a bit of oil and vinegar.

Nutritional Information per Serving:

- Calories 19
- Fat 1.4g
- Carbohydrate 0.3g
- Dietary Fiber 0g
- Net Carbs 0.3g
- Protein 1.5g

MOZZARELLA STICK SUBSTITUTE

Serves: 3

Preparation time: 25 minutes

Ingredients:

- 3 lemons
- 1 pound fresh mozzarella cheese
- 2 large garlic cloves, crushed
- ½ tsp. salt
- ½ cup olive oil

Fresh oregano and basil, finely chopped

Preparation: Heat a frying pan on medium heat and cut the cheese into long rectangles about 1/4th of an inch thickness. Squeeze the juice from the fresh lemons to get about 4 tablespoons of fresh juice. In a small bowl, mix the garlic and salt and then add the lemon juice to make a paste. Add the ½ cup of olive oil until you get a substance that has the consistency of mayonnaise. Toss the cheese batons in this mixture and then place on the frying pan and fry for 2 – 3 minutes, turning halfway through. Remove from the heat, place on a serving platter and sprinkle with basil and oregano before serving.

Serving Suggestion: A simple tomato marinara sauce is a great, low-carb dressing for these sticks.

Nutritional Information per Serving:

- Calories 286
- Fat 24.1g
- Carbohydrate 4.8g
- Dietary Fiber 0.9g
- Net Carbs 3.9g
- Protein 15.1g

STUFFED PEPPERS

Serves: 3-4

Preparation time: 25 minutes

Ingredients:

- 12 baby bell peppers
- 2 large ripe avocados
- 1 lemon, juiced
- ¼ cup cilantro, chopped
- 1 tsp. hot chili sauce
- 12 pieces of bacon
- Salt and pepper to taste

Preparation: Pre-heat the oven to 375°F and cut the peppers lengthwise into halves. Place on a baking sheet and bake for about 12 minutes until tender. While cooling, fry the bacon in a large skillet until brown. When cool, crumble the bacon and add to the mashed avocado flesh along with the lemon juice, cilantro, chili sauce and seasoning to taste. Fill the peppers with the avocado mixture and enjoy.9.

Serving Suggestion: Eat quickly as the hot mixture will make the peppers soggy if you try to save them.

Nutritional Information per Serving:

- Calories 141
- Fat 10.8g
- Carbohydrate 4.6g
- Dietary Fiber 2.6g
- Net Carbs 2.0g
- Protein 8.8g

QUICK AND EASY GUACAMOLE

Serves: 4

Preparation time: 10 minutes

Ingredients:

- 4 ripe avocados
- 2 tablespoons of freshly squeezed lime juice
- 1 small red onion very finely chopped
- Salt and freshly ground pepper to taste
- Paprika or a little cayenne pepper to garnish

Preparation: Cut the avocados in half lengthwise and remove the pit. Remove the flesh with a spoon a large glass bowl and mash with a fork. Add the rest of the ingredients and mix finely.

Serving Suggestion: This can be eaten by itself or served with any bread substitute.

Nutritional Information per Serving:

- Calories 106
- Fat 9.8g
- Carbohydrate 5.2g
- Dietary Fiber 3.5g
- Net Carbs 1.7g
- Protein 1.0g

ASPARAGUS AND HAM

Serves: 2

Preparation time: 15 minutes

Ingredients:

- 30 small spears of fresh green asparagus
- 12 slices prosciutto ham
- Olive oil with sprigs of rosemary

Preparation: Thoroughly wash and dry the asparagus spears and snap off the root end if too tough. Cut the ham and wrap around each asparagus spear. In a large frying pan, heat a little olive oil and fry the wrapped asparagus for about 5 minutes turning regularly. Serve hot for a great snack.

Serving Suggestion: This can also make a great meal when added to any bread substitute.

Nutritional Information per Serving:

- Calories 91
- Fat 4.7g
- Carbohydrate 3.1g
- Dietary Fiber 1.3g
- Net Carbs 1.8g
- Protein 9.8g

PORK SKINS

Serves: 3-4

Preparation time: 1.5 hours

Ingredients:

- 2 pounds pork skin with a good fat layer
- Fine sea salt

Preparation: .Preheat your oven to 325° and line a baking sheet with parchment paper. Cut the pork skin into thin strips and then run with the sea salt. Place the skin, fat side down on the prepared baking sheet and cook for about 1.5 hours. Break along the scored lines and serve.

Serving Suggestion: This is a high protein snack, so it is best to only eat this snack on a day when the rest of your protein intake has been low.

Nutritional Information Per 2 oz. serving:

- Calories 308
- Fat 17.6
- Carbohydrate 0g
- Dietary Fiber 0g
- Net Carbs 0g
- Protein 34.8g

BEEF JERKY FROM GROUND MEAT

Serves: 4

Preparation time: 1 hour

Ingredients:

- 3 pounds ground beef
- 3 tbsp. salt
- 4 tbsp. light soy sauce
- Olive oil
- Spices of your choice

Preparation: Mix the salt into the beef in a large bowl. Oil the base of two large deep baking sheets with olive oil and then press the beef into the sheets dividing it evenly between the two. It should not be more that ¼ inch thick. Season the beef with the soy sauce and other desired seasonings before placing in a low oven at 150°F. Leave to dry out overnight, or for about 10 hours, until the jerky has hardened. Pour off any fat that may have accumulated.

Serving Suggestion: Once cooled, break into acceptable slices and then place in plastic bag in the fridge. While this will take a long time to make, it can be stored in the fridge for a quick snack for months.

Nutritional Information per Piece:

- Calories 45
- Fat 2.5g
- Carbohydrate 0.2g
- Dietary Fiber 0g
- Net Carbs 0.2g
- Protein 5.5g

STUFFED MUSHROOM SNACK OR APPETIZER

Serves: 4

Preparation time: 20 minutes

Ingredients:

- 20 small mushrooms
- 2 cups of canned crab, tuna or salmon
- 3 tbsp. finely snipped chives
- 3 cloves of garlic crushed
- 1 tsp. finely chopped thyme
- 1 tbsp. mayonnaise
- Salt and pepper to taste

Preparation: Clean the mushrooms gently and remove the stalks and ribs. Pre-heat the oven to 375°F and lay the mushrooms on the baking sheet, top down. Drain fish or crab and mix it together in a bowl with garlic and herbs. Add the mayonnaise to moisten and season with salt and pepper to taste. Fill the mushroom caps generously and bake for 13 minutes.

Serving Suggestion: Consider serving these hot as the taste will be irresistible.

Nutritional Information Per mushroom

- Calories 31
- Fat 1.4g
- Carbohydrate 0.5g
- Dietary Fiber 0g
- Net Carbs 0.5g
- Protein 4.0g

BACON AND EGGS WITH A FLARE

Serves: 3-4

Preparation time: 20 minutes

Ingredients:

- 12 large free range fresh eggs
- 8 slices of bacon
- ½ cup mayonnaise
- 1 tsp. mustard powder
- 1 tbsp. powdered cumin
- Salt and freshly cracked black pepper
- Paprika for dusting

Preparation: After hard boiling the eggs, fry the bacon slices and drain excess fat with a paper towel. Crumble the bacon. Cut the eggs in half and scoop out yolks to add to the bacon. Add mayonnaise, mustard, cumin, and salt and paper. Mix together with the bacon and egg yolks. Fill the egg white halves, sprinkle with paprika and serve.

Serving Suggestion: These can be prepared ahead of time and be kept in the refrigerator for a quick snack throughout the day.

Nutritional Information per Half Egg Serving:

- Calories 80
- Fat 5.7g
- Carbohydrate 1.6g
- Dietary Fiber 0g
- Net Carbs 1.6g
- Protein 5.9g

Chapter 7: Top 5 Keto Soups and Salads

MACKEREL SALAD

Serves: 3

Preparation time: 25 minutes

Ingredients:

- 2 mackerel fillets
- 2 large eggs
- 1 medium avocado
- 2 cups green beans
- 4 cups mixed lettuce such as lamb lettuce, arugula, or kale
- 1 tbsp. ghee
- ¼ tsp. salt or more to taste
- freshly ground black pepper

For the lemon and mustard dressing, use:

- 2 tbsp. extra virgin olive oil
- 1 tsp. Dijon mustard
- 2 tbsp. lemon juice

Preparation: Hard boil the eggs. Cook the green beans for 4-5 minutes. Make small cuts on the side of the mackerel and season with salt and pepper. Heat a pan with ghee and add the fillets. Cook until the skin is crispy and brown. When the eggs are chilled, peel and quarter. Wash the lettuce and dry and place in serving bowl with green beans. Add eggs, sliced mackerel and drizzle with the dressing which is made by simply adding and mixing the three ingredients.

Serving Suggestion: You could switch the mackerel for any other type of fish you have.

Nutritional Information per Serving:

- Total Carbs 16.1 g
- Fiber 8.5 g
- Net Carbs 7.6 g
- Protein 27.3 g
- Fat 49.9 g
- Calories 609 kcal

CREAMY COLESLAW

Serves: 3

Preparation time: 20 minutes

Ingredients:

- 1 cup mayonnaise
- 1 tbsp. Dijon mustard
- 2 tbsp. apple cider vinegar
- 1 tsp. celery salt
- 1 tbsp. red onion, minced
- 1 large carrot, grated
- 5 cups green or purple cabbage

Preparation: Mix together the mayonnaise, Dijon mustard, apple cider vinegar, celery salt, and red onion. Add the vegetables and mix some more.

Serving Suggestion: It is best to let this refrigerate for 4 hours before serving.

Nutritional Information per Serving:

- Total Carbs 6g
- Fiber 4 g
- Net Carbs 2 g
- Protein 1 g
- Fat 28 g
- Calories 264

Simple Side Salad the Keto Way

Serves: 4

Preparation time: 15 minutes

Ingredients:

- 3 cups mixed greens
- 2 tbsp. extra-virgin olive oil
- 1 tbsp. balsamic vinegar
- 1/4 tsp. sea salt
- 1/2 medium avocado, diced
- 2 green onions, thinly sliced
- 2 tbsp. raw sunflower seeds
- 2 oz. chèvre, crumbled

Preparation: In a large bowl, combine mixed greens, extra- virgin olive oil, balsamic vinegar, and sea salt. Top with the avocado, green onions, sunflower seeds and chévre.

Serving Suggestion: If you don´t like vinegar, replace with lemon juice or even orange juice.

Nutritional Information per Serving:

- Total Carbs 11g
- Fiber 6 g
- Net Carbs 5 g
- Protein 10 g
- Fat 30 g
- Calories 330

HEARTY ITALIAN STEW

Serves: 3-4

Preparation time: 25 minutes

Ingredients:

- 1/4 cup extra-virgin olive oil
- 1/2 cup yellow onion, diced
- 1/2 cup carrot, diced
- 1 garlic clove, minced
- 1 lb. ground mild Italian sausage
- 1/2 medium green bell pepper
- 1 tbsp. tomato paste
- 4 cups chicken stock
- 8 green kale leaves
- 1/2 lb. kielbasa, sliced
- 1 tsp. Italian seasoning
- 1/4 tsp. crushed red pepper flakes
- 1/4 cup fresh basil, chopped

Preparation: Sautee onion, carrot and garlic until soft. Add the Italian sausage and brown for about 5 minutes. Add bell pepper and tomato paste and cook for 3 more minutes. Next, add the chicken stock, the kale, kielbasa, Italian seasoning, and crushed red pepper flakes. Cover and simmer for 30 minutes. Add salt if necessary and sprinkle with basil on top.

Serving Suggestion: This hearty soup goes great with Keto cracker substitute.

Nutritional Information per Serving:

- Total Carbs 12 f
- Fiber 4g
- Net Carbs 8g

- Protein 22 t
- Fat 45 g
- Calories 525

SEAFOOD CHOWDER THE KETO WAY

Serves: 4

Preparation time: 45 minutes

Ingredients:

- 1/4 cup unsalted butter
- 1/4 cup shallots, diced
- 1/4 cup carrots, diced
- 1/4 cup celery, diced
- 1/2 tsp. dried thyme
- 2 cups vegetable broth
- 1/4 lb celery root, peeled and diced
- 1/2 tsp. sea salt
- 1/ tsp. freshly ground black pepper
- 2 cups heavy cream
- 1/4 lb. live and cleaned clams
- ¼ lb. fresh salmon, cubed
- ¼ lb. raw scallops out of shell
- 1/4 lb. raw shrimp

Preparation: Heat up a soup pot Heat a large soup pot and add butter to sauté all of the vegetable ingredients. Next, add the vegetable broth and salt and pepper and simmer for 20 minutes until celery is softened. Stir in the cream and then add the clams. Simmer for 3 more minutes. Finally add the salmon, bay scallops, and shrimp and simmer for an additional 1 to 2 minutes, or until seafood is cooked through and clams have opened.

Serving Suggestion: You will want to serve this delicious, hearty soup immediately. Add Keto cracker substitute for dipping.

Nutritional Information per Serving:

- Total Carbs 12 g
- Fiber 1 g
- Net Carbs 11 g
- Protein 20 g
- Fat 59 g
- Calories 655

Chapter 8: Top 5 Keto Desserts

COCONUT AND ALMOND BITES

Serves: 3

Preparation time: 35 minutes

Ingredients:

- 2 large egg whites
- 2 tsp. raw honey
- 1 tsp. pure almond extract
- 2 cups unsweetened shredded coconut
- 16 whole almonds
- 4 oz. 85 percent cacao dark chocolate bar
- 1 tbsp. coconut oil

Preparation: Preheat the oven to 350°F (180°C). In a bowl, mix the egg whites, raw honey, and almond extract and coconut. Form this mixture around one almond to make a small ball. Add unsweetened coconut and mix until combined. Place on parchment paper lined baking sheet and cook for 12 minutes. Melt the dark chocolate and drizzle over the coconut bites.

Serving Suggestion: If you really love chocolate, you can dip the coconut bites into it instead of just drizzling it on top.

Nutritional Information Per Serving:

- Calories 268
- Fat 24g
- Protein 4g
- Total Carbohydrate 14g
- Dietary Fiber 5g

- Net Carbohydrate 9g
- Fat 81%
- Protein 6%
- Net Carb 13%

Cheesecake Muffins and Berries

Serves: 4

Preparation time: 40 minutes

Ingredients:

- 1.5 cups pecans
- 4 tbsp. unsalted butter, melted
- 1/8 tsp. sea salt
- 1 tsp. powdered stevia
- 24 oz. cream cheese
- 1.5 tsp. pure vanilla extract
- 2 large eggs, beaten
- 1 cup heavy whipping cream
- 1 tsp. liquid stevia
- 3/4 cup fresh berries of choice

Preparation: Preheat the oven to 350°F (180°C). Place pecans in food processor and then combine the crushed pecans, butter, sea salt, and the stevia mix. Divide the mixture into a muffin pan with muffin paper cups. Bake for 5 minutes. In a separate bowl, beat the cream cheese, vanilla extract and the rest of the stevia. Add eggs and beat lightly. Add this creamy mixture over the baked muffin crusts and bake for another 25 minutes. Before serving, add the whipped cream, liquid stevia and the rest of the vanilla extract. Add this mixture on top with a few berries to serve.

Serving Suggestion: Instead of serving hot, you might consider leaving these muffins to chill overnight in the fridge and serve cold.

Nutritional Information per Serving:

- Calories 422
- Fat 42g
- Protein 6g
- Total Carbohydrate 6g
- Dietary Fiber 1g
- Net Carbohydrate 5g

CHOCOLATE PEANUT BUTTER CUPS

Serves: 4

Preparation time: 20 minutes

Ingredients:

- 8 oz. 85 percent cacao chocolate bar
- 1/4 cup coconut oil
- 3/4 cup unsweetened peanut butter
- 2 tbsp. raw honey
- 1/8 tsp. sea salt

Preparation: Melt dark chocolate in double boiler along with the coconut oil. Add a bit of this chocolate mixture into lined muffin pan and freeze for 15 minutes. In separate bowl mix the peanut butter, honey and sea salt. Add the peanut butter mixture over the frozen chocolate and then add remaining chocolate mixture. Place in refrigerator for 2 hours before serving.

Serving Suggestion: You can top these scrumptious bites with some whipped cream if you prefer.

Nutritional Information per Serving:

- Calories 240
- Fat 20g
- Protein 5g
- Total Carbohydrate 13g
- Dietary Fiber 3g
- Net Carbohydrate 10g

MANGO AND COCONUT PUDDING

Serves: 3

Preparation time: 20 minutes

Ingredients:

- 1 400ml can full-fat coconut milk
- 1/3 cup white chia seeds
- 1 cup fresh mango, diced
- 1 tbsp. toasted sesame seeds

Preparation: Combine the coconut milk, white chia seeds, and mango and mix well. Cover and refrigerate for 8 hours or until gelled. Add toasted sesame seeds on top before serving.

Serving Suggestion: This recipe can also be frozen for a type of Popsicle.

Nutritional Information per Serving:

- Calories 299
- Fat 27g
- Protein 5g
- Total Carbohydrate 15g
- Dietary Fiber 6g
- Net Carbohydrate 9g

ALMOND TRUFFLES

Serves: 4

Preparation time: 60 minutes

Ingredients:

- 8 oz. 75 percent or higher chocolate
- 4 fl. oz. heavy cream
- 1 tsp. almond extract
- 1/4 cup unsweetened cocoa powder

Preparation: Chop chocolate into small pieces. Heat up the cream and almond extract stirring occasionally. Pour this cream mixture over the cut up chocolate pieces in a small bowl. Once the chocolate melts, spread a thin layer on a lined baking sheet. Chill in refrigerator for 20 minutes. Once cooled, roll the chocolate into individual small balls and coat these balls in unsweetened cocoa powder.

Serving Suggestion: You can either serve these immediately or place in the refrigerator to serve throughout the week as a delicious desert.

Nutritional Information per Serving:

- Calories 138
- Fat 12g
- Protein 2g
- Total Carbohydrate 8g
- Dietary Fiber 3g
- Net Carbohydrate 5g

Chapter 9: Top 5 Keto Drinks

PUMPKIN SMOOTHIE

Serves: 2

Preparation time: 20 minutes

Ingredients:

- 1/4 cup pumpkin purée, unsweetened
- ¼ cup almond milk, unsweetened or water
- ½ tsp. pumpkin pie spice mix
- 1 scoop whey protein powder (vanilla or plain) or egg white powder
- ¼ cup crème fraiche or sour cream or plain full fat yogurt or coconut milk
- 2-3 drops liquid stevia
- 1 tbsp. extra virgin coconut oil
- ¼ cup coconut cream on top

Preparation: Mix all the ingredients together in a blender. Top with coconut cream.

Serving Suggestion: This is a filling drink that is a great addition to a light breakfast.

Nutritional Information per Serving:

- Calories 399
- Fat 32.6g
- Carbohydrate 10.3 g
- Dietary Fiber 0g
- Net Carbs 6.7g
- Protein 21.8g

Vanilla Smoothie

Serves: 2

Preparation time: 10 minutes

Ingredients:

- 2 large eggs or 2 tbsp. chia seeds or 2 tbsp. coconut butter
- ½ cup sour cream or coconut milk
- ¼ cup whey protein or egg white protein powder
- 1 extra virgin coconut oil
- 1 vanilla bean or 1 tsp. vanilla extract
- 3-5 drops Stevia extract
- ¼ cup water + ½ cup ice

Preparation: Place everything into a blender. Pulse for a couple of minutes and serve immediately.

Serving Suggestion: While some people may not like the idea of eating raw eggs, you can purchase pasteurized eggs to calm any fears you may have.

Nutritional Information per Serving:

- Total Carbs 5.6 g
- Fiber 0.5 g
- Net carbs 5.1 g
- Protein 34.6 g
- Fat 45.2 g
- Calories 565 kcal

CHOCOLATE SMOOTHIE THE KETO WAY

Serves: 2

Preparation time: 10 minutes

Ingredients:

- 2 large eggs or 2 tbsp. chia seeds or 2 tbsp. coconut butter
- ¼ cup heavy whipping cream or coconut milk
- ¼ cup whey protein or egg white protein powder
- 1 tbsp. MCT oil or extra virgin coconut oil
- 1 tbsp. cacao powder, unsweetened
- 3-5 drops Stevia extract
- ¼ cup water + ½ cup ice

Preparation: Add all of the ingredients to the blender and pulse until well mixed. Serve immediately.

Serving Suggestion: If you want to cut back on the protein, simply don't add the whey protein or egg white protein powder.

Nutritional Information per Serving:

- Total Carbs 7.2 g
- Fiber 2.8 g
- Net carbs 4.4 g
- Protein 34.5 g
- Fat 46 g
- Calories 570 kcal

COFFEE THE KETO WAY

Serves: 2

Preparation time: 5 minutes

Ingredients:

- 1 cup brewed coffee
- 1 tbsp. extra virgin coconut oil or MCT oil
- 1 tbsp. unsalted grass-fed butter or ghee
- 3 egg yolks
- 1 tbsp. of gelatin, hydrolyzed which does not cause liquids to gel
- ¼ - ½ tsp. cinnamon
- 3-5 drops of stevia or a teaspoon of Erythritol or Swerve
- 2 tbsp. coconut milk or heavy whipping cream

Preparation: Place everything into a blender and blend until smooth.

Serving Suggestion: If you like your coffee hot, place in the microwave for 30 seconds before serving.

Nutritional Information per Serving:

- Total Carbs 4.4.g
- Fiber 1.3 g
- Net carbs 3.1 g
- Protein 15.2 g
- Fat 45.6 g
- Calories 474 kcal

Low Carbohydrate Cappuccino

Serves: 2

Preparation time: 5 minutes

Ingredients:

- 1/2 cup espresso
- ¼ cup coconut milk
- pinch cinnamon or raw cocoa powder (unsweetened)

Preparation: The trick here is to get the coconut milk to froth. Use a milk frother to make it bubbly and then heat it up. Add the milk to the hot espresso using a spatula to hold back the foam. The foam goes on the top allowing you to try your hand at making designs.

Serving Suggestion: You can add a few drops of Stevia sweetener if you like your cappuccino sweetened.

Nutritional Information per Serving:

- Total Carbs 2.4.g
- Fiber 0.7 g
- Net carbs 1.7 g
- Protein 1.3 g
- Fat 12.2 g
- Calories 133 kcal

Conclusion

Radically cutting back on your carbohydrate intake while simultaneously increasing the amount of meat and fat in your diet might seem like it goes against the commonly accepted nutrition knowledge. Since the time were in elementary school, we learn those famous nutrition periods that tell us that a healthy diet is one with limited fat and high carbohydrate intake.

Despite this fact, recent studies have shown that the Ketogenic diet offers numerous health benefits for a wide variety of people. Whether you are trying to lose weight, reduce the risk for heart disease, or simply feel more energized and mentally aware, the Keto diet can help you improve your health while also allowing you to enjoy a wide variety of great food.

Making the transition to a diet that is low in carbs might take a bit of getting used to. Our species has been growing and eating carbohydrates as the basis of our collective diets for thousands of years. However, with the guidelines outlined in this book along with the 60 complete recipes for meals, snacks, and drinks at all times of the day, the Keto diet will be easy to adhere to while you enjoy the numerous benefits that come with this unique diet.

22358608R00051

Made in the USA
San Bernardino, CA
11 January 2019